THE SIMPLE PLAN

DISCOVER HOW A FEW SIMPLE RULES CAN HELP YOU CONTROL YOUR INTAKE, PRIORITIZE AND LIVE A HAPPIER LIFE

AF808407

David Havens and Donald Morris

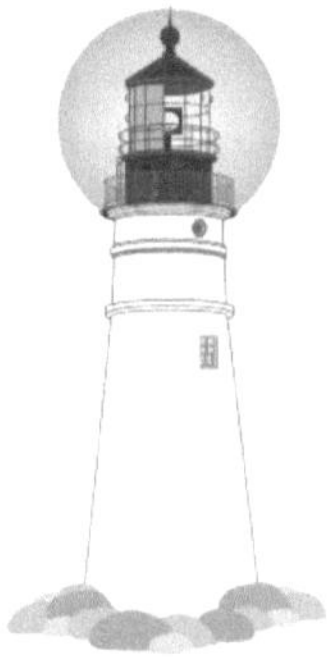

THE SIMPLE PLAN

DISCOVER HOW A FEW SIMPLE RULES CAN HELP YOU CONTROL YOUR INTAKE, PRIORITIZE AND LIVE A HAPPIER LIFE

David Havens and Donald Morris

ETA Solutions

Educate • Train • Anticipate

ETA Solutions

Educate • Train • Anticipate

Educating and ***Training*** today's leaders to ***Anticipate*** the next move.

www.buckeyefrog.com

Copyright © 2021 by David Havens and Donald Morris

All rights reserved. No part of this publication may be reproduced, stored in a retrieval system, or transmitted, in any form or by any means, electronic, mechanical, photocopying, recording, or otherwise, without prior written permission from the authors.

ISBN: 978-0-9982959-4-7

Book Cover and Graphic Designs by

David Havens and Donald Morris

Printed in the United States of America

Dedication

I'd like to dedicate my small contribution to this book to my mom and my sister. They both were taken way too early by the insidious disease of Alzheimer's. They were gentle souls who loved life and the beauty of the world around them.

I've observed that the vast majority of physical ailments we suffer are self-induced, mostly from what we consume, but also how we live life. This book is about taking control of your life through what you eat, the hours you sleep, and finally by keeping the goals you've set for yourself.

We consume processed foods, drink excessive amounts of alcohol, lack proper amounts of sleep, and most importantly, go through life with little or no direction or purpose.

My mom and sister had no choice in dealing with Alzheimer's disease. It just took them.

While scientists still do not know how to prevent or reverse Alzheimer's, they have determined factors that lessen the likelihood of having to deal with it. That is my purpose for this book.

If my contribution to humanity is that you set this book down and finally decide to improve how you live and **what you allow** into your life then I have succeeded.

Enjoy.

Don Morris

DISCLAIMER

Allergies and health situations should always be taken into consideration before beginning any type of dieting or intake program. Always consult a doctor, physician's assistant or certified nutritionist if you have any questions about dieting or how certain foods or fluids may affect your body or certain health conditions.

During any type of dieting or intake program always ensure you stay well rested and properly hydrated. If at any time you have questions or concerns consult a licensed physician.

The information that has been put together for this book is based on the personal experiences and opinions of the authors, including research, observation and common sense. The authors do not assume any liability, on any level, for the use of, or inability to use, any or all of the information included in this book. They also take no responsibility for any problems of any kind that may be incurred by the reader due to the information found in this book. Use this material at your own risk.

We the authors are not doctors. We're not scientists, human physiologists or certified nutritionists. We did our best to explain the science parts of this book while keeping it as simple as possible. We apologize if we missed a step or failed to fill in all the gaps, but the overall goal throughout the writing of this book was always to inform, to motivate and to provide a *simple* plan.

If you are that guy or gal that looks for the negative in everything in hopes of exposing the "Aha!" or "Gotcha!" moment, this book is probably not for you. This book is for those who are looking for a ***Simple Plan*** to move forward in life.

Table of Contents

Amphit For Life

SEAL Teams, also known as "frogmen," operate with an Amphibian approach that encompasses Sea, Air and Land (SEAL) in all types of environments. This Amphibian approach to operating is why we are also known as "Frogmen." You can develop an *Amphibian* approach to synchronizing your life for maximum productivity by building upon this method of operation. I call this being *Amphit For Life*. Being Amphit, which is my term for Amphibian fit, requires bringing together three items that make up a formula for success in life, Mind, Body and Intake or what I refer to as MBI. All three are essential and work together to ensure maximum output. This formula translates into Achievement.

MBI works just like the fire triangle. To keep a fire burning at optimum performance you need three things heat, fuel and oxygen. If one of these is lacking the fire will sputter and if one of them ceases to exist it will go out.

Likewise, maximum productivity will not be accomplished if the three elements of MBI aren't operating efficiently. If you have a positive mindset, but lack the health and fitness to climb a set of stairs without becoming winded you're falling short of your true capability.

If your health and fitness are dialed in, your brain is freed up to be as creative and solution-oriented as possible. When your health and fitness are lagging, your brain is unable to fully focus on the overall objective. Coming up with solutions to counter bad intake decisions or sending signals throughout the body to slow down in order to prevent injury or worse, preoccupies your brain and delays achievement.

The inverse is equally poor. I would say sometimes even worse. You can be fit and eat healthy, but if you are lacking a Front Sight Focused mindset the result will be the same, failure to reach your full potential. The mental and physical challenges of

Life have to be met with a Front Sight Focused Mindset, a fit Body and a controlled Intake.

Achievement starts with a Plan, is moved forward with Passion and is captured through Consistency.

A Note from the Author

When I retired from the US Navy as a US Navy SEAL I was at the top of my game, but the further I got away from my retirement date I found I wasn't winning the health and fitness game. To be more to the point, I wasn't winning the midsection game. I was working out twice as hard, but not getting the results that I felt I deserved for my time and effort.

It was several years later while training some operators from the Special Operations community that I discovered the knowledge that would form the basis of this book. At that time my go-to snack on the trail was trail mix and peanut butter. During a break from land navigation training, I took a jar of peanut butter from my backpack. As I began to open the jar of peanut butter one of the operators, who happened to be a Navy SEAL, made this comment; "If you read the book *It Starts With Food* you would never eat peanut butter again." Hearing those words from someone I didn't know may have enticed me to be a little confrontational with them or just blow them off, but because it came from one of my brothers, it got my attention.

We continued to discuss this in depth over the course of that afternoon. He told me to read the first part of the book where the authors explain each of the various food groups and how they affect the body. He added that the knowledge in that section alone is enough to change your life.

I went home after that event, ordered the book and when it arrived I read every word. I completed the 30 day *Whole 30* plan and it changed my life. The knowledge I gained, more than the results, is what blew my mind. I couldn't believe how wrong I was for all those years. I realized I hadn't taken enough time to really get into the weeds and do the research, and was surprised to learn that some of the nutritional information I had read and heard over the years was untrue. Before my encounter with *It Starts With Food* I would pride myself on my accomplishments due to my health and fitness knowledge. The reality, however, was my job was masking my results.

"What?"

I'll explain.

In the SEAL Teams working out is something that is built into your everyday work schedule. Normally the first two hours of your work day revolve around Physical Training such as CrossFit style workouts, running, obstacle courses, weightlifting, swimming and combination type events. These combination events mixed workouts with various aspects of the Navy SEAL job. A typical Friday combination event, aka *Monster Mash,* may involve a half-mile ocean swim, four-mile run with a rucksack, and another half-mile swim followed by an obstacle course and shoot and move drills using your primary and secondary weapons. Keep in mind these workouts were not just for staying in shape they were also for competition. Everything we did in the SEAL Teams was about winning the event or pushing for a personal best. Now couple that with the rest of your work day. This could be day and night dives navigating underwater for hours using a re-breather diving apparatus or jumping out of an airplane in full combat equipment, landing and patrolling for eight kilometers to go do reconnaissance.

Still with me?

I tell you this because the intense physicality of the job was giving me a false sense of accomplishment on the nutritional side of the house. It's easy to think you are eating healthy or that you have your nutrition locked up tight when you are shredded and maintaining good size and strength.

Reality Check: When your job or daily activities burn high calorie numbers it's easy to fall victim to this illusion. If you have a job or a lifestyle like this you can make bad intake decisions and get away with it for a period of time, but here is the problem. If you don't have the knowledge and take precautions when you transition from that lifestyle to a much slower one your choices are going to catch up with you …with a *quickness*.

I always felt like I was going 100 mph when I was at the top of my game in the SEAL Teams, but as soon as I retired I was only going a 100 mph during my daily workout. The rest of my day I was only doing the speed limit or less. Couple this with my slower metabolism due to age and my eating habits, which remained at pre-retirement levels, and I was destined to get only one result. I was no longer winning the body fat game.

I consider myself lucky that I went as far as I did before I was hit with the realization of how this game works. My job and my lifestyle at the time were the only reasons I was winning for so long. I would say most people experience this realization a lot earlier in life, probably around age 30 and I'll tell you why.

During high school most of you were involved with sports or other similar activities that can fix most intake decisions. This activity level combined with a youthful metabolism makes it easy to navigate these waters.

Following high school you start college or you enter the work force. Even if your activity slows down slightly during this period of time, it is still a pretty forgiving period due to your metabolism. You are likely the intern, the junior sales person or the one stuck taking care of all the odd jobs, which means you are probably the most active person at your work place. Even juggling marriage, kids, career and a metabolism that is starting to ebb you can still be winning without making too many changes to your diet.

I'm not a doctor or nutritionist by any means, but I would say around the ages of 25-27 a new variable begins to come to the forefront, *Stress*. Believe it or not, your decline in the game usually begins with a promotion. More responsibility means more time stuck at your desk, more time spent sitting in meetings and possibly more stress from worrying about losing your job if you don't perform well.

This means less activity to help with burning those extra calories.

I would say age 30 is where you start to really notice who the winners are in this game. For some of us you may have seen this as early as your 10 year high school reunion. Like it or not, metabolism doesn't get better with age. To be able to start putting W's back in the *Win* column you have to start controlling your intake.

The information in this book is not a compilation of new health discoveries or part of a new dieting trend. It's a simple, easy to follow, set of guidelines for anyone from beginner to expert.

I've taken what I have learned over the last five years and cleaned it up so knuckleheads, like myself, can read and understand it. I've simplified it for longevity. I did this for one reason. I want you to *Achieve*.

David Havens

Introduction

The S.I.M.P.L.E. Plan is designed to right the ship and get you back on course. What we're about to explain is a system of basic fundamentals that will set the foundation for you to start moving forward towards a healthier You.

Your body is like a ship. From the outside it looks pretty simple, but on the inside it can be a little overwhelming. The nice thing is, once someone shows you around it's about as *simple* as finding the bathroom in your house. I'll let you in on a little secret. There are very few things in life that are impossible. With most things, once someone pulls back the curtain and eliminates the "knowledge is power" variable it loses its mystic. The same is true with human physiology and how your body handles the things you intake.

The S.I.M.P.L.E. Plan gives you a blueprint for a strategy that is not only simple and easy, but can be integrated into almost any lifestyle.

The older we get the more our ship starts to list due to changes in our metabolism, less and less daily activity and bad intake decisions, that include food or fluid. These are the facts of life that come with age, work and raising a family.

When an actual ship is listing or leaning to one side, it can still continue to operate and in most circumstances it can still complete its day to day functions. The problem is it's not an efficient way to do business. In order to remain operational, adjustments have to be made to the timeline and procedures have to be modified. Continuously operating in these types of conditions can, and in most cases, cause problems over time. When unexpected situations present themselves, such as bad weather things can escalate.

Now here's the beautiful reality to this scenario, there is a solution. All you have to do is right your ship! This is achieved by balancing out the load and controlling what's being taken onboard, which is your intake. This is how the body is designed to work. You have to balance out your lifestyle, Mind, Body and Intake.

By implementing the S.I.M.P.L.E. Plan we are going to show you how to balance out your intake and clean up your decision making process. This can be done by just following a few S.I.M.P.L.E. guidelines or what we call in the SEAL Teams Standard Operating Procedures (S.O.P.s).

It's never too late to start developing a healthier eating mindset. By changing a few things in your normal routine you can immediately start to balance out your ship. Controlling your intake will put you back on offense and allow you to start moving the ball down the field.

Now before we continue, I need you to slow down.

"What?"

This is the point where I imagine a lot of people would start thinking about gym memberships or downloading the latest dieting or fitness App. There is no need right now to start worrying about exercise, meal plans or measuring out food. I'll even go you one better. At this point in the game I'm not even interested in counting calories. Before we can venture down that path you have to understand and master the initial S.O.P.s involved with Sleep, Space and Schedule.

Remember this*, All is never lost.* This is the mindset that is necessary if you want to continue moving forward in life and achieve your objective. Think about this when it comes to controlling your intake. You've made it this far in life even with all of the bad intake decisions you have made over time, like overeating, alcohol, excessive sugar or binging on your favorite comfort foods. It's never too late. We've all made mistakes or what I call a *mess* when it comes to the subject of intake. The S.I.M.P.L.E. Plan puts the ball back in your court so you can take the steps needed to start winning.

A key to your success is to implement this plan without upending your lifestyle. This is accomplished by using the *Crawl, Walk, Run* approach. Whenever you start something new in life you first need to crawl, then stand up and walk, and once you feel like you have control you can take off running. This system is not rocket science, not even close. It's a simple plan that anyone can use to start moving forward.

One of the reasons people lose motivation after they start something new is because they take on *too much too quickly*. Changing your eating habits or starting a new workout without a well thought-out plan can easily get overwhelming. This in turn can lead to excuses that propel a downward spiral into what eventually results in quitting. The S.I.M.P.L.E. Plan is a system specifically designed to prevent you from taking on *too much too quickly.* Preparation and consistency coupled with a good plan always sets the stage for success.

The S.I.M.P.L.E. Plan is built around three principles designed to help you achieve and maintain your goals:

The plan has to be simple and efficient; not only easy to learn, but easy to do. It has to make sense and be able to be easily added into your everyday lifestyle.

The plan has to produce results in a relatively short period of time. For the majority of people that means literally seeing results.

> When people look in the mirror they are only thinking one thing, "Show me the money." I know I don't have to say this, but I'm going to, *people are impatient.* We are living in the Amazon generation where most things in life are only a click away from being delivered to your house. The same is true with any type of eating plan. Everyone expects results…NOW!

The plan has to be easily explained. People like to talk about what they are doing and to show off their results, both in person and on social media. To do this it has to be easily explained and be believable.

If you can't explain it to an eighth grader, you don't understand it well enough.

Intake

A healthy lifestyle starts with developing an ability to control your intake. A controlled intake sets the stage and feeds your capacity to succeed in all areas of your life.

A controlled intake, with healthy choices, fuels the creative process in the mind and builds motivation through inspiration that comes from achieving results. Good intake also helps with the body's immune system and preparing it for the daily stresses of life and repairing it afterwards.

This system doesn't bring anything new to the table. This book doesn't bring to light any new glaring discoveries. It doesn't need to. Basic human physiology works pretty much the same for everybody. I know there are exceptions, but I'm not in the exceptions business I'm in the reality business. The reality is this; you can begin to right the ship at any time you want. It is easier when you are younger, but if you are willing to put in the time and effort all is not lost.

What we've done is set up some simple rules (S.O.P.s) that make up a foundation that can lead to success. These are easy to follow guidelines that if followed with consistency can produce amazing results.

This intake approach is not designed to be the know all, end all. This system is a set of guidelines to get you moving in the right direction, so you can legitimately start managing your own situation. Getting back up on step, starts with having a good plan. A good intake plan starts with a dialed in Front Sight Focus mindset, research/knowledge and simplicity. If an intake plan is too strict or has too many rules it's going to be difficult to sustain over a long period of time.

"Is it even possible to maintain super strict programs over a long period of time?"

The short answer is "Yes," but it takes special people and special situations to navigate these waters. The majority of these special situations revolve around extreme health conditions or specific professions related to physical performance which usually lead to big payoffs $$$.

This system is strict in nature, in that you have to stick to the plan, but it is built around a common sense approach. It's more about following a few simple rules and building from there. Depending upon your overall goals you can amp it up or tone it down to achieve your desired result. Not everyone has the same health and fitness goals in life. Some people spend their whole life without ever setting foot inside of a gym. That's ok. It's more about your health than it is about how many workouts you get in or miles you run per week.

"So how does it work?"

The S.I.M.P.L.E. Plan is made up of five categories that make up the acronym that titles the book. Each letter in the word *simple* represents one of the five categories that drive the overall plan. For the plan to gain momentum and move towards success each one of these will have to be followed and for it to have longevity each one will have to be mastered.

The “S” in the S.I.M.P.L.E. Plan is made up of three items Sleep, Space and Schedule. These items make up the initial load plan that puts us on a course for righting the ship. I call this the S3 shop because it reminds me of the S3 section on a Battalion Command Staff in the US military. The S3 is responsible for the Battalion’s training and all operations during combat. This section also anticipates situations that may present themselves and prepares contingencies using unit S.O.P.s to mitigate them.

The same is true with the body. Sleep, Space and Schedule (S3) are responsible for laying the initial foundation to run operations. The S.O.P.s involved with establishing the S3 give the brain, the digestive system, the pancreas and the liver the best chances for mitigating all intake decisions.

CHAPTER 1

Sleep

"Early to bed and early to rise makes a man healthy, wealthy and wise."

–Benjamin Franklin-

"Sleep? I thought this was a book about what you put in your body."

Even though we like to think fueling the body is just a food and fluid thing, it's actually made up of two different items. Food and fluid being one part and sleep as the other. Believe it or not you need one just as much as you do the other. Actually, after reading the book *Why We Sleep*, by Matthew Walker, PhD, I'm beginning to think sleep may just be a little more important.

I'm not going to let the cat completely out of the bag, but Walker outlines some pretty sobering facts. I have highlighted some findings from the first chapter that drive home not only the importance of sleep, but give you an overview of how sleep can balance out your life and feed your success. Conversely it can also hold you back from achieving your true capability if the correct daily amount is not being received.

There is no denying sleep play's a major role in assisting the immune system, but it cannot be understated how it affects your metabolic state and assists in balancing blood sugar. Maintaining good blood sugar levels aids appetite control, which in turn helps you make better food decisions. Those better food decisions can help with your micro biome in your gut which can lead to better nutritional health.

All major organs, including your brain, benefit from a full night's sleep and can be negatively impacted when sleep is cut short. Messing around with your sleep can also contribute to major conditions such as depression, anxiety and suicidality.

Walker makes a strong case that sleep deprivation increases your risk of cancer and operating in that state over long periods of time can play a role in whether you develop Alzheimer's disease. Adequate sleep combined with exercise and healthy eating habits provide a platform for the best long-term health outcomes.

In his book Dr Walker lays out a good plan for navigating these waters. He recommends following his *Twelve Tips for Healthy Sleep* from the National Library of Medicine's *Tips for Getting a Good Night's Sleep.*

Here is an overview of what he suggests:

Establish a sleep schedule. Start a routine before you go to bed so your body is prepared to go to sleep. If possible get up around the same time each day.

Don't exercise or consume caffeine too close to bedtime. For some people caffeine can take up to eight hours to leave the system. This goes for nicotine too. Nicotine can cause light sleep which hinders the healing effects of sleep, so it should be avoided late in the day as well.

Heavy alcohol use can also have the same negative affect causing lighter sleep and preventing good REM sleep. Alcohol can also affect your breathing, which can hinder sleep and cause you to wake up intermittently.

Don't eat large meals late at night or consume too many fluids close to bedtime. Indigestion can result from eating too much too close to bedtime and too many fluids can cause you to wake up to go to the bathroom at various times throughout the night.

Some medications have side effects that can cause sleep disruption or contribute to insomnia. If your medicine is preventing you from getting a full night's sleep consult your physician about possible alternatives.

Avoid late afternoon naps. A hot bath before bed can help you relax and in some cases help you fall asleep more quickly.

A cool, dark room free of blue light gadgets makes for a better sleeping environment. Sometimes watching the clock can prevent you from falling to sleep. Dr Walker suggests turning the clock face away from you to prevent worrying about the time.

Take in the sunlight. Get outside at some point during the day and feel it on your face. Believe it or not this helps with regulating your sleep schedule.

If all of the above aren't working and you still have trouble sleeping, then get out of bed and do something relaxing, like reading, until you feel tired. This can help prevent anxiety from not falling asleep on time.

A good trailer for *Why We Sleep* is Joe Rogan's podcast episode #1109. The guest for that episode is Matthew Walker PhD.

Nothing works in life without good, quality sleep. Understanding this and implementing it is paramount on any path leading to success. A good eight hours of sleep is what allows you to operate at your true capability; producing ideas and enhancing creativity. Sleep drives the train. Like I said before, knowledge is power and in this game sleep gives you the power to succeed.

To better understand the benefits of sleep and the details involved I highly suggest reading Dr Walker's book Why We Sleep *Unlocking The Power Of Sleep And Dreams.*

CHAPTER 2

Space and Schedule

"Schedule and Priorities should go hand in hand"

-David Havens-

When it comes to integrating health and science, learning is best achieved when the information is broken down to a beginner level.

Surprise, surprise, right?

So, for example, let's imagine your body as a distribution center. This center has a large building with multiple loading docks, where vehicles arrive and unload packages of all shapes and sizes. Let's say these packages represent the food you eat.

When everything is running smoothly and operating as planned the system runs as a well-oiled machine. When vehicles show up, packages get unloaded, sorted and sent to their correct destinations without any problems or delays.

In the shipping industry a key variable is *time*. It takes a certain amount of *time* to ship an item to a distribution center, unload it, sort it and transport it to its final destination.

During holiday seasons such as Black Friday and the weeks leading up to Christmas the company has mechanisms in place to hire extra people to ensure packages arrive at their destinations on time. Despite this planning, complications can also happen and shipping can slow due to unforeseen circumstances.

A similar version of this occurs in the body. You eat a meal (packages arrive), and the various components of protein, carbohydrates and fat get digested (unloaded and sorted) and moved to their assigned locations.

During this natural process if there is too much food being taken onboard, or in some cases not enough food, the body uses the pancreas to send out signals to store the extra or pull some out of storage to meet the demands of the body.

In the shipping industry this is the equivalent of hiring part-time workers or laying people off to ensure the company remains productive and profitable.

This is how the system works in a perfect world and in that world it requires *time*. Time is what makes this work.

Now let's move back to the shipping scenario. Everything is moving as scheduled when all of a sudden unscheduled vehicles start showing up at the distribution center. These extra vehicles have unknown amounts of parcels onboard. In the short term, such as holidays and big events, the company can flex work schedules with overtime or hire part time help, but what if it starts happening all the time, on all the shifts? What if the times that they show up are always random and the volume of shipments are always different? The company would need a bigger building, more loading docks and more personnel in hopes of possible mitigation. If there was no method to the madness, and it was always random, it would lead to an indefinite amount of chaos and problems.

In the body these unscheduled deliveries are eating between meals. When you normally finish eating your body comes up with a solution for taking care of what was consumed at the meal. It calculates a plan and the amount of time it needs to complete it.

When you intake unscheduled items they have to be put someplace. These storage areas look a lot like your waistline, your hips/thighs and your chin. When these unscheduled or not needed items get excessive they can lead to the far worse consequence of negative health conditions.

The key word here is *time*. When we translate *time* into S.I.M.P.L.E. Plan terminology this is known as *Space*. *Space* is a major part of the equation as our body requires time to do its job and help us achieve our ultimate goal of good health. This is not rocket science. Not even close. This is basic human physiology. Your body has only so much time to offload items and get them to their final destination. Anything extra doesn't fair well.

"Space? What does that even mean?"

You have to put space between your meals. When I refer to *space* I'm talking about not eating between meals; no snacks, no sodas, no nibbling on anything. This space is only for hydrating. To be more specific I mean water only. Sounds strict, but it's paramount to establishing the initial foundation that drives the system. Space will always be the one variable in the formula that resets the switch any time life happens to get in the way. You're not always going to be perfect every day of the week. That's ok. Space is the reset button.

"How long is this space between meals?"

Five hours.

"Why five hours?"

To explain this let's go back to the beginning where I said this plan is designed to prevent you from taking on *too much too quickly*? A key goal is to minimize thoughts of giving up or quitting.

The objective (don't quit) and longevity rule number one go hand in hand. Longevity rule number one states:

"It has to be simple and efficient; not only easy to learn, but easy to do. It has to make sense and be able to be easily added into your everyday lifestyle."

The key word here is *lifestyle.* The wrinkle is we all have different lifestyles and they're built around a plethora of different things, such as culture, ambition, gender, religion, mood… The list is endless. To tackle this dilemma of *space* you have to identify an amount of time that will naturally fit into the majority of everyone's lifestyle. This means you need a common denominator that fits into most everyone's normal daily *schedule*. Five hours accomplishes this without upsetting your daily routine. The funny thing is this time variable of five hours has been around since the industrial revolution. The sad part is, over the past 30+ years, we've done just about everything we can to remove it from our daily schedule. Through the acceleration of daily life, the easy access to fast food and the over consumption of snacks we've managed to erode away this historical standard. To some consumption looks more like one gigantic meal that stretches from the time you get up to the time you go to bed. In case you were wondering, in our opinion, there is no such thing as a healthy snack when it comes to your body.

"What?"

There is no need to eat between meals unless you have a legitimate health problem, such as Diabetes.

In order for this to work we have to agree that there are three meals in the day, breakfast, lunch and dinner. You can call them whatever you want, but the plan calls for three. The plan also calls for you to eat all three meals. You can argue all you want, but rules are rules.

"I don't eat breakfast. Why is eating all three meals so important?"

I don't have a case study to give you that proves this, but common sense sometimes has to step in and point out the obvious. Your body is an amazing system that works 24/7. Fueling it whenever you feel like it doesn't pass muster. To maximize your body's full potential and to do this effectively your daily intake needs to be evenly spaced across your waking hours. Fueling it efficiently is the best formula for ensuring success.

Ok, here's why five hours makes the best time variable. Using a traditional work day, let's say you get up in the morning around 6:15am. You brush your teeth, shower and get dressed. Around 6:45am you make breakfast and you finish eating around 7:20am. Now it's off to work to start the day. Next on the list is lunch.

What time do most people normally go to lunch?

12:00 o'clock?

Ok, if we give ourselves some time to walk to the lunch room or in some cases drive to the nearest restaurant were probably starting lunch around 12:20ish. If we do the quick math on that scenario 7:20am to 12:20pm …ish is five hours. By the time we finish eating lunch it's probably getting close to 1:00pm and it's back to work we go. Next up on the list is dinner time.

Once we get off work we head home, pick-up the kids, go to soccer practice or run errands. When we finally arrive home for dinner it's probably getting close to 6:00pm. You're probably already ahead of me in this scenario and know what's coming next. You guessed it we're at five hours again.

Now I know this timeline is the "perfect world" scenario, but it is based on a traditional work *schedule*. Is it going to happen like this every single time? No, it's not. Sometimes life gets in the way, but here's the thing. In the real world the times might move slightly to the left or right, but we have a plan and the plan has a schedule. When obstacles arise switch to contingency mode and figure it out. Come up with a solution and mitigate.

"So... how does that work?"

Sometimes the meals aren't going to be eaten in the lunch room or at your dining room table. This is reality speaking. Sometimes you have to swing through the drive thru, that's life. I'm going to keep repeating this one phrase, "All is not lost every time it doesn't go as planned." When you get off schedule take a deep breath, reset, re-assess and Charlie Mike (Continue Mission). The five hour time variable is going to be our reset button throughout this whole system. Initially, it's not about what you're eating it's about the frequency of your eating. We need to establish the S3 foundation and master it before we start attaching the rest of the S.I.M.P.L.E. Plan components.

"That's it?"

Almost.

There is one other key that goes along with this schedule. This last S.O.P. is what holds the S3 foundation together. After the dinner meal there is no more eating until breakfast the next morning. You read that correctly. Once dinner is complete eating for the rest of the day is over. I know this can be tough. This was the hardest thing for me and it wasn't because I was legitimately hungry later in the evening. It was because I had to break the habit of my nightly visits to the pantry. My evening routine included eating a snack while I watched Netflix or finished up something from work. The hours from dinner to bedtime can be brutal because these nightly patterns have been engrained into us over time. Monday Night Football and movie night are the worst, but here is why this S.O.P. is so important. The five-hour space between meals is to allow your body to clean up the meal you just ate and honestly there are times that some meals may not have been the healthiest choice. In those situations your body may require more than five hours to do its job. The extra time that you collect en route to breakfast allows the body time to work on leftovers from those bad intake decisions. The quicker we master the S3 plan the sooner we can be on our way to righting our ship.

I was in my mid-forties when I started implementing the S3 S.O.P.s. It was rough, but within a couple of weeks I started experiencing real results. Not only results I could view in the mirror, but the ones I could feel too. I was sharper and more creative. I could feel my body starting to right itself and begin to stay up on step longer. With my stamina more predictable it allowed me to be more productive throughout the day. When your body can count on you to give it the best advantage to win your results are going to be nothing short of amazing.

CHAPTER 3

Intermittent Fasting

"The best of all medicines are resting and fasting."

-Benjamin Franklin-

In an article written for healthline.com Kris Gunnars defines intermittent fasting as "an eating pattern where you cycle between periods of eating and fasting."

"And what is fasting?"

When you look up *fasting* on Google it defines it as "abstaining from all or some kinds of food or drink, especially as a religious observance." In a more detailed search Google goes on to say; "Fasting is a deliberate abstinence from physical gratification, usually going without food for a period of time, to achieve a greater spiritual goal. Fasting is intentionally denying the flesh in order to gain a response from the spirit."

I'll be straight up with you. I dread the actual word. When I hear the word *fasting* the only thing that enters my mind is "Ugh." And, for the most part, I think the majority of us have the same feeling whenever we hear anything that has to do with it. For years it was something that stayed pretty close to the religious side of the house and only occasionally ventured into other areas such as medical procedures involving surgery or having your blood drawn.

I don't want to waste a lot of time drifting around all the different types or ways to conduct intermittent fasting, but there are benefits. In his article Gunnars identifies some pretty compelling evidence that aligns with a number of other findings, studies and claims. Here are some of the benefits that top most lists and are included in the Gunnars article:

-Calorie control

-Metabolism boost

-Effectively lose weight and belly fat

This information sometimes makes me laugh because of the amount of truth it holds. If you aren't eating you aren't taking in calories. It's that simple. It may seem funny, but once you step back and analyze the information you will soon realize, it's basic human physiology.

Intermittent fasting or putting space between your meals, i.e. controlling your intake, does have other benefits other than just losing weight.

In an article on hopkinsmedicine.org titled *Intermittent Fasting: Is It for You?* the author,

Karen Nitkin, talks about research data that indicates intermittent fasting offers many benefits including lowering blood pressure and cholesterol as well as losing weight. She also writes about its effect on Parkinson's and Alzheimer's disease and decreasing the risk of cancer.

That information alone should be enough to get you moving in the right direction, but wait there's more.

Intermittent fasting can help reduce insulin resistance and lower blood sugar levels.

"What is insulin resistance and what does it have to do with blood sugar?"

Hmmmm…well, I knew this day would come. Once you venture down this road long enough it's eventually going to intersect with questions about blood sugar. I never really liked science and I definitely don't like teaching it, but it's important. Scratch that. It's beyond important. It's the entire ship, the captain, the engineer, the quartermaster who plots the course, the person who stands watch on the bridge wing and the guy in aft steering.

Understanding blood sugar and insulin resistance is how you begin to set yourself up for the best chances of long-term health. The tricky part is explaining it, *simply*. I covered a general overview of it with the shipping and distribution analogy I used in chapter 2, but to get the full effect of why insulin resistance is so bad I'm going to have to add to it and dare I say it, I'm also going to have to use some real science terms. "Ugh."

Alright, let's get to it. When doctors, nutritionists and trainers talk about blood sugar they are referring to the measured amount of glucose (sugar) in the blood. Your blood circulation is the primary transport system for distributing vitamins, nutrients, oxygen and water to the various cells throughout your body.

When you intake food and fluid your body's digestive system starts to break it down so you can use it as fuel. Different types of food and drink can affect your blood sugar differently. These affects can be from the amount you intake as well as how quickly that food and drink can be broken down for transport in the blood stream. I don't think I need to explain how the amount portion of that statement works, but the latter part may be of interest. Enter the Glycemic Index.

Don't worry I didn't know how it worked either until a few years ago.

This science gem is rather important when it comes to blood sugar, especially if you have diabetes. In 1981 Dr David Jenkins, a scientist at the University of Toronto, and some of his colleagues developed a scoring system for grading how fast food can be broken down and converted to glucose.

Here's how it works. The index grades food on a scale of 1 to100. If an item has a score of 100 it is pure glucose. The index is split up into three categories low (1-55), medium (56-69) and high (70-100). Some examples in the high category are white bread (71) and baked potato (85). Oatmeal (58), banana (62) and white rice (64) fall into the medium group. Whole grain pasta (42), apple (39) and broccoli (15) are on the low end.

Now that you understand how the Glycemic Index works it's easier to understand the difference between simple and complex carbohydrates. Simple carbohydrates breakdown quickly into glucose (sugar) while complex ones take longer.

To appreciate why this is so important you have to understand what glucose does and why it is imperative that you keep it regulated properly. Glucose is the primary source of energy for the body's cells and it's also the main source of fuel for the brain. It is imperative that the level of this vital fuel be kept stable. High blood glucose over long periods of time can damage the kidneys, eyes, nerves and other organs. It can also increase your risk for heart disease, heart attack and stroke.

The glucose in your blood is regulated by the two hormones insulin and glucagon. These two hormones are produced in the pancreas and are used to keep your blood glucose in homeostasis or stable.

Insulin's job is to decrease your blood glucose levels and glucagon's job is to increase it. These two hormones work in conjunction to keep your blood glucose levels balanced.

When your blood sugar increases, like it does right after you eat, beta cells in the pancreas sense this and stimulate the pancreas to release the hormone insulin into the blood stream. This tells the body cells they can absorb glucose and it can also signal muscle cells and the liver cells to take on glucose and store it as glycogen. Insulin's job is to act as a key to unlock the cells to absorb glucose or take it on and store it as glycogen.

When your blood sugar is low alpha cells in your pancreas sense this and stimulate the pancreas to release the hormone glucagon to act on the liver to break down the stored glycogen into glucose to be released into the blood stream to elevate blood glucose levels.

The Centers for Disease Control and Prevention says that within two hours of eating your blood sugar levels should return to normal. The blood sugar numbers work like this; 140mg/dL or lower is considered normal two hours after eating, 140 to 199mg/dL indicates pre-diabetes and 200mg/dL or higher indicates you have diabetes. You would need to see a physician to confirm the latter.

Too many calories and constantly eating in between meals can cause your blood glucose levels to remain high over a longer-than-normal period of time. This can lead to insulin resistance and sometimes much worse, diabetes.

When you are insulin resistant your cells don't respond to insulin like they should. The insulin key no longer works well at unlocking the body's cells, which causes an excess build up of glucose in the blood and can lead to pre-diabetes. When this happens the cells don't have their fuel necessary to do their jobs. This in turn causes the pancreas to try and send more insulin to fix the situation, which only causes a higher insulin state in the blood. When there is high insulin in the bloodstream it can be difficult to burn fat. When you have a high insulin state it can also encourage fatty acids that are floating around in the blood to go into fat storage. When you're insulin resistant your energy level will be low, you will have carbohydrate cravings and weight gain is right around the corner.

"How do you fix it?"

You right the ship by controlling your intake with better decisions, staying active and exercising and getting proper sleep. Sleep deprivation can cause your cells to be less sensitive to insulin so make sure you are getting eight hours of sleep a night. A combination of cardio and resistance training is an effective way of increasing insulin sensitivity. Exercise helps move sugar into the muscle cells for storage, which can cause an immediate increase in sensitivity that helps keep your blood glucose levels under control. Controlling your intake and making good carbohydrate choices can give your body more time to regulate your blood glucose levels. This is easily accomplished by using the Glycemic Index.

Reducing your stress and losing excess weight can also increase insulin sensitivity. There are also two other key things that can help you get a jumpstart on ensuring you have the best chances of staying away from becoming insulin resistant.

The first one is *space.* By understanding how blood sugar works and what is involved with keeping it stable you can start to appreciate the full meaning of adding space between your meals. Space affords your body time to clean up and regulate the amount of sugar that is in your blood stream so your body can perform.

The second thing can be a little more difficult, but at some point in the game minimizing added sugar has to be addressed. Minimizing added sugar is a game changer, but I'll be the first to admit this is easier said than done.

"Why is that Captain Dave?"

The answer is simple. Almost everything you enjoy eating or drinking has added sugar. Having said that, I used the word "minimize" for a reason. We want to eliminate added sugar, but we still need to approach this change through the crawl, walk, run process. I think most people know where their shortfalls lie when it comes to their intake issues. If I was guessing I would say the majority of these issues revolve around sugar.

"I don't have a sweet tooth."

That may be true, but we need to understand that sugar doesn't just come from chocolate, sweets and ice cream. This fact brings us back to that "knowledge is power" thing. Most of the time, our problems with sugar come from eating between meals and consuming too many carbohydrates such as bread, cereal, pasta, rice and sugary beverages. The sleeper among these is the sugary beverages. For example, a 20 oz. Mountain Dew has 77 grams of sugar. To break that down so everyone can understand just how much that is in the big sugar picture--it is 19 teaspoons. That translates to a little more than 1/3 of a cup of sugar. That's crazy! You can control your eating intake all you want, but if you are guzzling sugary beverages like Mountain Dew, Coke or Gatorade, throughout your day, you're not even close to being in the game. Added sugar is the enemy. If you couple this consumption behavior with the inability to control your food intake you can add even more variables.

Eliminating added sugar is the goal, but it's not going to happen overnight. For most of us, sugar has been a big part of our intake for most of our lives. If we want to achieve this objective and want to maintain it for longevity we have to wean ourselves down to an acceptable amount and go from there.

The key is to monitor your calories, make healthy intake decisions and put space between your meals. There are a lot of advantages from abstaining from eating, but it should only be done if it doesn't upset your eating schedule and your daily lifestyle.

We believe the S.I.M.P.L.E. Plan has intermittent fasting already built into the schedule. It's designed with two five hour windows and another that averages around 12 hours. That's almost 22 hours of not eating. I don't know how much more fasting you need to do. This plan allows for meal time windows to be on schedule and evenly spaced over your waking hours as well as providing your body the time to perform and function in the way it was intended.

There are all types of strategies to enhance your health, but controlling your intake with the S.I.M.P.L.E. Plan and staying active with a Front Sight Focused mindset is always going to be a winning combination.

When you add it up, it becomes apparent that the proper blend of *Sleep, Space* and *Schedule* that's included with the S.I.M.P.L.E. Plan affords you a solid solution.

CHAPTER 4

Minimize

"Efficiency of time and efficiency of effort starts with unloading the unnecessary."

-David Havens-

Let's talk about calories for a minute. I know there is all kinds of information floating around out there. Some of it is good and some of it is partial facts mixed with random conversations, social media posts and dieting myths. To keep it simple it basically works like this. If your calorie intake count is higher than your expended calorie count that comes from activity and metabolism, you are not going to lose weight. If you burn more calories than you intake you are going to lose weight overtime. You can argue quality vs quantity of calories all you want, but in the end it is about numbers in vs numbers out. I know there are rare exceptions in the game, but I'll reiterate for all the naysayers. I'm not in the exceptions business. I'm in the reality business and the reality is you have to be accountable to yourself.

If you have a rare condition, then seek a professional to help you come up with a solution. More times than not, I find that the "condition" which seems to get easily classified as "hereditary" normally is missing an official diagnosis from a doctor. Stop making excuses. If the goal is to lose weight and the plan is to track calories to accomplish this then you should probably measure everything you eat. A little extra here and there makes a difference in the big scheme of things. Just because nobody is around to see you take an extra bite or add another scoop doesn't mean it didn't happen. You are not going to fool your body and your digestive system. They catch everything. And here is the bonus that most of us forget about. Other things such as sleep and when you are eating can help you win the overall health equation.

Having said all that, I need to add some caveats before we continue. It is true that keeping track of your calories in and your calories out is a technique for gaining or losing weight, but that technique alone is not one that I would recommend or consistently use overtime. This brings up the calorie quality argument.

"A calorie is a calorie."

Yes it is, but what is the objective? Most of the time, the overall goal is to lose, gain or maintain your weight. The overall goal of the S.I.M.P.L.E. plan is to do this efficiently while maintaining good health and immunity. To do this requires good *Sleep*, *Space* and *Schedule* and controlling the quality of your intake.

"So what does that look like?"

Controlling our *Sleep, Space,* and *Schedule* is what helps us adjust our load plan so we can get organized and begin to start moving forward through these waters. To continue this momentum for the long haul and to do it efficiently we need to learn how to adjust for tides and currents. In the intake world this is learning how to *minimize* bad intake decisions.

Your body only needs a certain amount of calories to support your daily activities. Any extra calories get processed and sent away to storage. Storing extra calories leads to increased body fat and too much body fat leads to eventual health problems.

There are ways to prevent these stores from getting too big. One of them is activity, which translates into cardio and resistance training. The other way is through control which brings us back to that calorie thing. The key is maximizing the quality of these calorie numbers to ensure the overall goal is being met.

"Figuring out calorie intake and how this process works makes my head hurt."

My only response to that comment is "yeah it can be a little overwhelming," but I have good news.

Michael Matthews hits this head on in his best-selling book Bigger Leaner Stronger. He breaks it down into 3 *simple* steps.

1. Calculate your Basal Metabolic Rate (BMR)

2. Calculate your Total Daily Energy Expenditure (TDEE)

3. Calculate your target daily calorie intake

"I don't know how to do any of that let alone how to calculate it. I don't know what any of those terms even mean."

Slow down! Not to worry. This is why we titled the book The S.I.M.P.L.E. Plan. There is something you learn early on in the SEAL Teams that is also relevant in everyday life, work smarter not harder.

In his book Matthews also includes a link to a free calculator on his website that does all of this math for you with the click of a few buttons. He has figured out the formulas and built them into the calculator. You can find the calculator tool at the following link:
www.biggerleanerstronger.com/calculator

Before you run off to use this link let me share with you some simple knowledge of how a calories in calories out system works. Understanding BMR, TDEE and how these numbers help develop your target daily calorie intake establishes the next level in your progression. Once you master *Sleep*, *Space* and *Schedule* (S3 SOPs) the next phase of your advancement is cleaning up your meal intake decision making process. Effectively spacing out your macros (protein, carbohydrates and fat) and the number of calories for each is what ensures efficiency.

The data being entered into this calculator is only half the battle. Knowing what to do with the results is the game changer. The calculator itself uses formulas that produce numbers based off of your inputs. In order to maximize the effectiveness of the results you need to understand how it all ties together.

"Ok, what is BMR?"

BMR stands for Basal Metabolic Rate. Your BMR number is the number of calories that your body burns while it's at rest. In other words it's how many calories your body needs to function if you didn't do anything. If you were just lying on the couch all day long you would still need a certain amount of calories to fuel your body. Calories are the fuel that runs your basic bodily functions such as brain activity, digestion, breathing etc. Identifying your BMR calorie number is the first step in understanding how to calculate how many calories you need to reach your overall goal of losing, maintaining or gaining weight.

Total Daily Energy Expenditure (TDEE) is the number of calories you expend from all of the activity you do throughout your day. This number is important because everything hinges on it. The BMR calories have to be met in order to keep everything running. TDEE calories are the ones that determine the success of the plan. Your TDEE is your BMR plus all energy expenditure that comes from physical activity and the energy involved with digestion and the processing of the food you eat. If the plan is to lose weight then you have to intake slightly less calories than your TDEE total. To maintain your current weight you try and keep your total caloric intake close to the total of your TDEE. Gaining weight works the opposite way as losing weight. To gain weight your daily caloric intake needs to be slightly higher than your TDEE total. The speed at which you lose or gain weight is dependent upon how much your daily caloric intake is over or under your TDEE.

"How much over or under is a good number for gaining or losing weight?"

In his book Matthews says there are studies that show cutting your TDEE calorie intake to 75% works well for both fat loss and muscle preservation when combined with resistance training and high protein intake.

On the subject of weight gain Matthews uses his experience and knowledge in suggesting you increase your intake to 110% of your TDEE calories to maximize muscle growth while minimizing fat gain. Having spent more than 30 years training and competing in fitness related events ranging from bodybuilding, triathlons and SEAL training I believe these numbers are on point.

"Ok, when it comes to protein, carbohydrates and fat how do I figure out how many calories should come from each?"

Also included in his book is a quick reference guide that lays out these percentages and shows you the formulas to use if you want to calculate a custom model for yourself.

This is what his macro calorie percentages look like for the basic goals of losing, maintaining or gaining weight.

	Lose Weight	Maintain Weight	Gain Weight
Protein	40%	30%	25%
Carbohydrates	40%	45%	55%
Fat	20%	25%	20%

During my research for this book I reviewed multiple websites to test various calculators and compare results. The calorie results for each of the categories BMR, TDEE and Target Daily Calorie Intake based on the goals to lose, maintain or gain weight were relatively close. What I found was the Bigger Leaner Stronger calculator was easier to use and easier to understand.

Why do I bring that up?

I bring it up because at the end of the Bigger Leaner Stronger calculator it also has a button that breaks down what percentage of those calories need to come from protein, carbohydrates and fat. It does this based on your overall objective to lose, maintain or gain weight. I really have to hand it to Matthews. His calculator is a one stop shop for quickly calculating the numbers you need to know to get moving in the right direction, but the thing I appreciate the most is its *Simplicity*.

"What's the next step?"

We've just talked about the basics of calories and how to calculate the number you need in order to continue moving towards your objective. Over time more and more of these calories will need to start shifting towards the quality side of the house.

I'm not going to sugarcoat it. This is where we're going to start tightening up the plan. This is where you decide if you are going to navigate these waters with accountability.

I want to reassure you. It is still a simple plan and it is still easy to understand. I know it can be a pain in the butt to start heading down this road and for some of us it's not the first time. From this point, the road is going to start to narrow, but it only narrows because it leads to success.

"How do I know what calories are good and which ones are bad?"

This is where I suggest homework for the naysayers and I share my food list with those who don't need to be convinced. That's not exactly true. The homework is for both of you. The food list is for those who want to keep it simple and easy.

Every time someone asks me what I'm doing to maintain the shape I'm in at age 51, I always tell them the same thing. I give them the Sleep, Space and Schedule elevator pitch and I finish it with this piece of knowledge, the *homework.*

If you really want to understand food and how it affects your body go get the book *It Starts with Food* by Dallas Hartwig and Melissa Urban and read pages 24-178. I do this for one reason. I'm not going to waste my time answering "What do you eat?" type questions for people who don't have any skin in the game.

Even though you, the reader, bought this book, which in essence gives you skin in the game, I still recommend the homework reading assignment. *It Starts With Food* breaks down all of the various food categories and gives you the good, the bad and the ugly. It dispels the myths and bad reporting that runs rampant throughout our society. It's an absolute knowledge game changer.

In this next section I'm going to walk you through how to put together the information from this chapter into a plan that is easy to learn and easy to do. To keep this simple I'm going to start this process by using the Bigger Leaner Stronger calculator. This will show you where to begin, how to figure out your intake numbers and what to do with those results. I'm going to do this by showing you my calculated numbers and how I use them to evenly space my food over my meal schedule.

Ok, let's do this.

Here are my numbers that I entered into the calculator and the accompanying results:

Question #1 "What unit would you like to use?"
Imperial (lb)

Question #2 "What's you gender?"
Male

Question #3 "How much do you weigh?"
168

Question #4 "How tall are you?"
5'9"

Question #5 "How old are you?"
51

Question #6 "How much do you workout per week?"

A moderate amount

(4 to 6 hrs of exercise per week)

Question #7 "Do you want to . . .?"
Maintain the same weight (Maintain)

Once you click on your choice for question seven the calculator tabulates your calorie results for the next two categories.

Your basal metabolic rate (BMR) is . . .
1612

Your total daily energy expenditure (TDEE) is . . .
2418

To **maintain the same weight**, you should consume the following calories and macronutrients every day: **2418**

When you click question seven it also tabulates the final section in the calculator based off of your answer to question seven.

30% of those calories should come from protein which amounts to 181g

45% of those calories should come from carbohydrates which amounts to 272g

25% of those calories should come from fat which amounts to 67g

The final three pieces of information that are provided at the end of the calculator are my favorite results. These are the numbers that make it all come together. The last three numbers tell you what percentage of those calories need to come from protein, carbohydrates and fat. It also breaks it down into how many grams you need for each.

Once you have these numbers you can spread them out evenly across your meal schedule so you can maximize your body's best chances of functioning more efficiently throughout the day. The next step in your progression will be the process of starting to crawl toward cleaning up each of these meals so you can maximize your calories en route to the overall objective.

Before we get into my food list let's talk about these numbers real quick. My question seven answer produced a total daily calorie intake of 2418 calories. This is what I need to take in to achieve my goal of maintaining. The results below it provide the blueprint for accomplishing this in the most efficient way. In a perfect world you would just take each of the numbers for protein, carbohydrates and fat and divide them by three for breakfast, lunch and dinner and call it good. The problem is it's not a perfect world and each item you purchase is not always going to be the exact same size and weight each time.

I'm not going to tell you that you have to weigh everything for every meal day in and day out. What I will tell you though, is when you initially start you should weigh everything to familiarize yourself with what each portion size looks like and go from there.

The list below is the items that make up the majority of my food list week in and week out. I do have to warn you it is a minimalist list. When it comes to sugar, dairy, bread, rice, beans and pasta I tend to stay away from them. I'm not going to say I never eat those items, but I try and limit my intake. After you read the homework assignment you will have a better understanding of why I choose to control my consumption when it comes to those items.

*The nutritional information below was acquired from multiple sources to include nutrition labels on product packaging and website databases.

Dave's Food List and Nutritional Information

Protein Items	Calories	Protein	Carbohydrates	Fat
4 oz Chicken Breast	124	26.1g		1.4g
5 oz Tuna Wild Caught	140	30g		2g
4 oz Lean Turkey Burger	230	19g		17g
4 oz Grass Fed Ground Beef	200	22g		11.2g
1 egg	71	6.3g	.4g	4.8g
Carbohydrate Items				
5.3oz Yellow Potato	110	3g	26g	
4.9 oz Red Potato	123	3.2g	27g	.2g

4.9 oz Russet Potato	134	3.68g	29.6g	.2g
6 oz Sweet Potato	105	1.9g	24.5g	.1g
5.5 oz Banana	89	1.1g	22.8g	.3g
6 oz Fuji Apple	95	.3g	23g	.3g
1 cup Blackberries	62	2g	14.7g	.07g
1 cup (1.1 oz) Spinach	7	.9g	1.1g	.1g
7 oz Green Pepper	33	1.4g	7.6g	.3g
4.5 oz Onion	48	1.1g	11.6g	<1g
3 oz Kimchi	24	1.5g	3g	

Fat Items

1 Tbsp Olive Oil	130			14g
1 Tbsp Coconut Oil	120			14g
2 Tbsp Cashew Butter	190	4g	9g	17g
7.1 oz Avocado	321	4g	17.1g	29.5g
1 Tbsp Ghee	45			5g
2 Tbsp Primal Caesar Dressing & Marinade Avocado Oil	130			14g

Supplements

Kirkland Signature Protein Bar (Costco)	190	21g	4g	7g

Fluid and Hydration

When it comes to fluids and staying hydrated I try and drink a gallon of water each day, but to achieve this goal takes a real conscious effort. I'll be the first to tell you I'm not always successful, but the goal is always there. In the morning I also normally drink two cups of coffee following my breakfast.

The following meal plans are examples of how I distribute my calories and macro totals (protein, carbohydrates and fat) throughout my daily meal schedule. I've also included one of my supplement meals with the meal plan examples. I occasionally use a supplement meal when I'm traveling or as a contingency if I think I may be running short on time.

Meal Planning

Breakfast	Calories	Protein	Carbohydrates	Fat
(6) Egg Whites (2) Yokes	210	27	1.6	10.6
11.5 oz Russet Potato	314	8.86	71.3	
1/4 Green Pepper	8.25	0.35	1.9	0.075
1/4 Onion	12	0.275	2.9	
(3) Cups Raw Spinach	21	2.7	3.3	0.3
(1) Cup Blackberries	62	2	14.7	0.7
(2) Tbsp Ghee	90			10
Total	717.25	41.185	95.7	21.675

Lunch	Calories	Protein	Carbohydrates	Fat
8.5 oz Chicken Breast	263.5	55.5		2.975
11.5 oz Russet Potato	314	8.86	71.3	
1/4 Green Pepper	8.25	0.35	1.9	0.075
1/4 Onion	12	0.275	2.9	
(3) Cups Raw Spinach	21	2.7	3.3	0.3
(2) Tbsp Ghee	90			10
(2) Tbsp Primal Kitchen Caesar Dressing	130			14
6 oz. Fuji Apple	95	.3	23	.3
Total	933.75	67.985	102.4	27.65

Dinner	Calories	Protein	Carbohydrates	Fat
10 oz Wild Caught Tuna	280	60		4
11.5 oz Russet Potato	314	8.86	71.3	
1/4 Green Pepper	8.25	0.35	1.9	0.075
1/4 Onion	12	0.275	2.9	
(3) Cups Raw Spinach	21	2.7	3.3	0.3
(1) Tbsp Olive Oil	120			14
Total	755.25	72.185	79.4	18.375

Supplement Meal	Calories	Protein	Carbohydrates	Fat
(2) Kirkland (Costco) Protein Bars	380	42	8	15
Fuji Apple	95	0.3	23	0.3
Banana	89	1.1	22.8	0.3
(1) Tbsp Cashew Butter	95	2	4.5	8.5
Total	659	45.4	58.3	24.1

Now that you have seen how I space out my calculated numbers throughout my meal schedule you can follow suit with your foods of choice and start developing your own meal plans.

Always remember this. Knowledge is power, but if you don't use it, if you don't action it, it's just words. I mentioned this earlier and the reality still remains. None of this is rocket science, not even close. It may seem foreign, but it's basic human physiology. It's how your body works and understanding this gives you all the power.

CHAPTER 5

Prioritize You

"Life Hint: You control the list. If it's a priority then move it up."

-David Havens-

We all prioritize our lives already. Take brushing your teeth for instance. You get out of bed, walk into the bathroom and one of the first things you do is brush your teeth.

Why?

Well, we know the importance of good dental hygiene so we make sure to brush first thing in the morning. Your toothbrush and toothpaste are right there in front of you. You don't have to go looking for them. You just reach out and put some toothpaste on a toothbrush and brush. Automatically. You don't even have to think about it. You probably have even been using the same brand of toothpaste for the last ten years. Automatically.

Think about it. Why is it so automatic? You spend no brainpower doing the same thing every morning. It's because that little act of dental hygiene is part of who you are. It is part of your identity. Think of it as your Self Image, your SI.

Our SI controls everything we do in our day. Everything we think, say, feel and do. Everything! It's the little small voice that talks to us all day long. It empowers us or many times holds us back.

I won't go into the psychology behind our SI. There are plenty of books written on the subject and rest assured, it is there controlling our every thought.

Picture a Hula Hoop. It's green. You are holding it about waist high. Unlike a traditional plastic one it is sturdy, like unbreakable steel cable, and it goes wherever you go throughout your day. You walk out of the bedroom in the morning and it is right there surrounding your waist. Climb into the car and it's with you. At work, at your desk, yup, it's still there. When you are talking to a boss or customer, again, it's there.

Funny thing is this green Hula Hoop represents our SI. Remember, your SI controls what you think and how you react.

For instance, you finally decide you want to lose some weight and you'll do it by running every morning. When the thought of working out enters your mind your SI starts giving you reasons it would be impossible. You're not a runner. It will take too long to get there. You'll look stupid. What if you hurt yourself? And on and on it goes.

Your Self Image is telling you who you are and what you can do and can't do. Right now, it is telling you, you are not a runner so get that out of your head.

But what if you resolve to get up the next morning and run? You set your alarm clock and go to bed. The alarm goes off at 6am just as you set it and you roll over and think to yourself, no way, I'm too tired. Next morning rolls around and you somehow force yourself to get out of bed and lace up your shoes. You open the back door and it's raining…nope, not today.

Your SI is controlling you. It will never let you stray far from the safety of the green Hula Hoop. It is your comfort zone. Oh, you can step outside of it maybe even get both feet outside of the green circle. But understand anytime we try something new and step beyond the circle our SI, our green circle, is always there to pull us back inside.

Whether you see yourself as an introvert or an extrovert, lean and fit or overweight it's your self-image. It's what you **believe** about yourself. We ALL have it. From the least to the most accomplished person we know. The person who seems so confident and has it all together carries his green Hula Hoop around with him wherever he goes.

I put the word **believe** in bold for a reason. I did this because the interesting little secret about that green Hula Hoop, seemingly made of steel cable, is that it can likewise act like a rubber band. It can be stretched and even enlarged permanently…if you know how to control it.

Oh, it's there and it's strong, because you **BELIEVE** it is strong.

Remember how I started this chapter with you brushing your teeth. You see yourself as a person who practices good dental hygiene.

You might be thinking right now, “but it’s brushing my teeth, there’s no effort in that.” Right. That’s because it is a part of who you are and what you do every morning. There are a hundred other little things you do throughout the day that are a part of how you see yourself. You buckle your seatbelt…or don’t. You salt your eggs…or don’t. You’re late to work every day…or not. It is all a part of how you see yourself.

So, the question is, why can’t we seem to stick with the things we know that would make us a better person? Things like healthy food decisions, or what we “spend our time thinking about” decisions, and even personality decisions.

You name it. The world is available to you and what you want to accomplish is only limited by your imagination.

You might not be able to be a starting wide receiver for a pro football team or a prima ballerina at the Met, so there might be SOME limitations. Those are minor compared to what else is yours simply for deciding and then taking action to move toward the positive changes you want.

OK, if it is so simple then what do you have to do to, let's say, run a mile non-stop? Oh, and you've never run a mile in your life and think those who do are nuts.

Your SI tells you that it's just not who you are, but you recognize it would be a healthy choice and are open to giving it a chance.

You start by defining what you want to accomplish. Then ask yourself, if I attain this what positive impact will it have on me and those around me? Write it down and post it on your mirror in the bathroom or slip it inside your wallet if you want to keep it to yourself. Then give yourself a reasonable deadline to accomplish it.

Want to run that mile? Then maybe 3 months is a reasonable timeline. Put it on the calendar and work backward noting what points you feel you should be at by certain dates.

Now for the fun part and I do mean fun!

You already know you won't want to get up in the morning and go run because it looms too large in your mind. The effort, pain, and oh, it might be raining!

To overcome these roadblocks you start by doing what I call **reducing it to the ridiculous.**

Can you set your alarm clock and get out of bed and put on your running shoes? That is it. That will be your absolute minimum you have to do every day, no matter what.

Can you do that? I'm pretty sure most people can.

"But wait, how is that getting me to a mile?"

Patience.

We are dealing with that green Hula Hoop that you carry around and we need to not let it know what we are doing. So again, can you wake up 30 minutes earlier and lace up your shoes? If you said yes then you are on your way.

By getting up earlier and doing this you are starting to change your Self Image. Remember, this is your absolute minimum. No matter what, you have to get up and lace up your shoes. Some mornings you might want to climb back into bed. Fine, but at least you did the minimum.

Here is the magical part. Some mornings you will say what the heck, I already have my shoes on I can at least go for a walk or a slow jog. And you will. Some mornings you will only get your shoes on. That is counted as a success! As you continue to build that habit (expanding your green circle) you will start to find it easier to get out of bed. Eventually that walk will become a slow jog or maybe a walk-run-walk.

If you are following your calendar then it will give you some motivation to beat that 3-month time frame you set for yourself. The very act of accomplishment that comes from lacing up your shoes every morning will start to feed off of itself and become its own motivation.

So back to the little secret about that green Hula Hoop. It is yours to control and you get to decide the size of it. It is always going to be with you, but by taking tiny ridiculously small steps you can accomplish many desired achievements. You will be able to do those things you always wanted to do, but could never find the time and made every excuse not to accomplish.

The other funny thing about your SI is that once you take control and start building your own SI it will seem odd to not make the good choices. To not workout will seem weird. To not choose nutritious food will seem odd. To not turn the TV off and read or learn something new becomes choices out of your comfort zone.

Does this mean you will never have another slice of birthday cake or simply sit and lose yourself in a mindless Netflix series? Not at all. The difference is you are now mindful of what you are doing. You are controlling what you eat and what information you allow into your world.

"So it's that easy? I just decide what I want and slowly start to move toward it?"

Yup pretty much! Why make it harder than it has to be?

I know what you are thinking right now. You are thinking well, I've tried to _______ (fill in the blank), but I have ___________ (name the excuse), so I just gave up and went back into my comfort zone, my happy little green Hula Hoop.

I mentioned earlier, there is a whole lot of science behind how we act and think and why we behave the way we do, but this is the essence of how to improve who we are and move toward positive outcomes to make our lives better.

Human kind, since we became self aware, has always wanted fuller, better lives. Whether it is embodied in the basics like food and shelter or higher-level needs like love and self-fulfillment; men and women are wired to want to control their lives.

To summarize and keep it *Simple*:

1. Decide what you want (a positive outcome).
2. Ask yourself, "What positive impact will this have on my life and those around me?"
3. Write down the desired outcome and the expected positive impact.
4. Break down the process to get there to the very basics. The step-by-step process working backward from you desired outcome.
5. Decide what is the absolute minimum you can commit to every day without exception.
6. Make it a priority.
7. Take action.

In fact, set this book down, pick up your phone and put your desired outcome into the notes section right now. Add the items I just listed and commit to start immediately with the absolutely most ridiculous small first step. Something you know you can commit to doing even on your weakest day.

Want to strengthen and accelerate the process? Identify a positive influence in your life who you can report to on a daily or weekly basis. Make it someone who won't find fault with your dream, but someone to hold you accountable. Just knowing you will have to show progress will add to your resolve to stay on track.

If you decide to do this, you need to be careful in your choice. Many times those closest to us are bad choices. They may see your positive change as a threat to their own green Hula Hoop. They are comfortable with you just the way you are because it validates their shortcomings. If you were to make changes such as losing weight, stopping smoking, or going back to school to get a degree, they may feel left behind. They could possibly find ways to sabotage your dream. Better to go it alone than have someone who will consciously or unconsciously undermine your success.

By the way, from this day forward, every time you pick up your toothbrush and squeeze out some toothpaste you will be reminded of the green Hula Hoop. It will be a daily reminder that you are in control of your life. You will be in charge of what you think and how you react to the events of the day. You are in control.

Toothbrush and toothpaste = Green Hula Hoop that you now control. Go buy a green toothbrush to help reinforce it.

CHAPTER 6

Live Life

"You are the only one holding you back and guess what? It probably started with your ears."

-David Havens-

Living life in the health and fitness world can be scary. It has its fair share of narcissists, alphas and yes, some crazies. These individuals usually present themselves in the form of the food police, fitness fanatics who never shut up and the liars that spew fitness myths. If I was guessing I would say it's what holds a lot of people back from starting any type of diet or beginning a fitness program.

To be successful and establish longevity as you're moving toward a healthier lifestyle you need the knowledge and freedom to live life guilt free.

Some plans use cheat days as a way of living life while on a diet or fitness regimen. I'm not a big fan of having cheat days. If you have a designated cheat day it's still a day that is in the schedule so if life hits you with something unexpected you're down a cheat day plus that period of time (# of meals) for whatever momentarily bumped you off schedule.

In order to live life guilt free you need the freedom to make adjustments on the fly. It may not seem like a big deal, but deep down your psyche is going to take a hit when you go off track and this is especially true if you have been knocking it out of the park. Even the most hardcore will feel a slight tinge of guilt, however small it may be, because they momentarily got off course.

Get rid of the cheat day. There is no need for it. The word itself, *cheat,* has a negative connotation. Instead call them unscheduled events. You know how to reset. When unscheduled events or situations in life happen you still need to keep moving. You still need to eat. Don't waste time stressing about it. Take a look around, assess the situation, identify your options, good or bad, and make a decision. Don't dwell on it. If McDonald's, Taco Bell and Wendy's are the only things in sight during a meal time-window then have it. If you're doing the best you can then all is not lost. It's an unscheduled event. Enjoy the meal. The real work is maintaining the space between the meals. With the freedom to make course changes en route to your objectives you will find yourself naturally starting to clean up your decision making process.

There is also another component of living life. Holidays, birthdays and special events, such as graduations, weddings and retirements should always be celebrated. Remember this little morsel. Christmas is not what put those extra pounds on you. The fact that you couldn't turn Christmas off until you were halfway through January is the real reason. When extended events, such as holiday seasons, start to appear on your horizon, have no fear. Instead, concentrate on being the Operations Boss of your S3 shop. *Prioritize* your *Sleep, Space* and *Schedule,* first, then adjust from there. When special occasions arrive enjoy them right along with everyone else. Eat and drink what you want, but try and keep the majority of your intake to meal times and adjust from there. Living life is paramount. It's what unites friends and family and creates lasting memories. Living life is what creates freedom and freedom ensures the best chances for health success.

This game is played with big boy/girl rules. You can justify anything you want to qualify as a special event, but you're only ambushing yourself if you're not being accountable.

Occasionally you may feel a need to create an unscheduled event such as taking the kids for ice cream or suggesting pizza night so you don't have to cook. Don't dwell on it. It happens. Sometimes you need a break. Try and keep decisions like this close to your meal time-windows in order to protect the space between your meals. If you can't so be it. Enjoy the event then reset, re-assess and Charlie Mike (Continue Mission). The big take away from this type of situation is to avoid this from turning into a habit.

When unscheduled events happen, don't forget to take some time to do a personal After Action Report (AAR). An AAR identifies what went wrong, tries to figure out why it happened and comes up with solutions to fix or prevent it from happening again. Sometimes there is nothing you could have done. If this is the case, own the events and move on.

Quitting is the only thing that secures Failure. If you're not quitting then don't call it a failure. Call it an obstacle. If you're going back to the drawing board to come up with solutions to mitigate then failure should never be in the conversation.

Don't forget that the Crawl, Walk, Run approach is key to your successful game plan and the longevity necessary to achieve your objective.

Living life in the S.I.M.P.L.E. Plan world needs to be exactly that, *simple*. I realize this new way of operating is probably going to clash with some of the things you have heard about or tried in the past. Once again, it's going to be Okay. We're going to crawl until we reach a point where we can start standing up and then we're going to start walking. Walking builds confidence and sets the stage for us to begin a slow jog which eventually leads to running. True running only occurs with experience. Experience is the only thing that prepares you for the unknown, the stressful situations, contingencies, emergencies etc.

Once you have some experience under your belt you can start to use this to your advantage when situations or opportunities present themselves. The more experience you have the easier it is to *anticipate* the next move. Once you have mastered the ability to *anticipate*, you can begin to side step life's potential hazards, predict opportunities, game plan effectively and win!

Initially your inspiration may have been generated by watching or reading about someone else's feats or accomplishments. As you move from short-term goal to short-term goal while graduating through the Crawl, Walk, Run process, your experiences and achievements will start to take over as your inspiration to continue the quest. You and your accomplishments, your health and fitness transformation, become your own motivation. There is nothing better in this game than the transition of your initial inspiration to becoming your own inspiration as a direct result of your own achievements. This transition will boost your motivation and confidence by leaps and bounds as you continue to gain momentum in the pursuit of your own objectives.

CHAPTER 7

Execute With Consistency

"Consistency is the act of revisiting the action over and over until you capture it."

-David Havens-

For the most part this book gives the appearance that your decision making process, when it comes to intake, is the most important thing, but there is an implied task that accompanies the process. If you aren't familiar with what I mean when I say implied task I'll explain.

In the military, operations begin with task orders in the form of specified tasks that state the various parameters and objectives of the mission. If it was a target intelligence package it would identify the target and the mission objectives, it would provide a history of intelligence reporting and layout a support package that would be available to assist with mission planning and execution. It may also include time parameters that must be adhered to, to ensure the best chances for success. From the specified tasks the team leader would infer what implied tasks needed to be accomplished in order to meet the specified tasks, the requirements of the mission objective.

"What?"

I'll give you an example of some implied tasks.

Let's say you are in combat and the mission objective is 50 miles away from your Forward Operating Base (FOB). Right from the beginning some of those implied tasks may include ensuring you have air assets standing by, during the operation, to provide a Quick Re-action Force (QRF) to assist in emergency situations. Having personnel with specific qualifications needed to fulfill certain mission requirements would be another. This could be as simple as ensuring qualified snipers are available for over-watch/security, qualified breachers for the assault team and a Corpsman to take care of any possible casualties. With time and distance being a major part of the equation, having food, water and medical supplies pre-staged for re-supply could also be on the list.

In the real world you might call this a *Given.* In today's society I think a lot of us have forgotten what that actually means. I bring this up because the *Implied Task* or the *Given* in the S.I.M.P.L.E. Plan is *Consistency.* In order for this plan to work…NO, change that. I need to re-word this so that it is clear, crystal clear. In order to ensure the success of the plan as a whole you have to Execute with Consistency.

"But how do you stay consistent over time?"

Every person is different in what drives them. What works for me might not work for you, but one thing is for sure. You need to identify what motivates you and make it your driving force. It may be one thing or a combination of things. Whatever it is it needs to be important enough to kick you in the backside and remind you of this when obstacles present themselves. For some it may be tied to family, for others it could be linked to money, dreams or power. I don't make the rules, but in order to achieve any of this there is one common denominator, good health. This is what ensures the best chances for long-term success. Living life with good health and prioritizing what is important to you, ensures longevity for whatever you choose.

CHAPTER 8

Conclusion

"Quitting is not an option."

-Everyone Who Has Ever Succeeded-

You picked up this book and you made it this far. You're almost finished. That says something about you as a person. You can finish what you start. Do not let anyone tell you otherwise. You are en route to greatness, period! This has to be your mindset. No excuses, complaining or whining. It is that S.I.M.P.L.E.

You are well on your way to establishing your *Day One*, the one that leads to achievement. You know the specified tasks that are required to ensure mission success. All you have to do now is identify the implied tasks and start moving (crawling) forward towards the objective. As you move along your timeline always remind yourself to keep it simple. When obstacles arise, switch to solution mode and figure it out. Don't overthink it.

Focus on your SI. Concentrate on expanding the size of your green Hula Hoop. Positive outlook as a whole feeds every aspect of your life. If you have to break it down to the ridiculous then do it.

To ensure longevity, over time, couple your movement forward with *Passion* and *Accountability.* True passion is the fuel that drives the train. When you see and feel results from your time and effort it's like filling up the gas tank and hitting the accelerator.

Always remember to use this fuel efficiently. This is done by being accountable to yourself and the loved ones around you. This is your health we're talking about. Having passion is one thing, but it only lasts so long if you aren't seeing results. I'm just being honest with you. You have to be accountable for your actions. When I was in the SEAL platoon we had a saying that went like this; "Don't be that guy." That goes for girls too. Don't be that person that holds up the train. Accountability and consistency go hand in hand in streamlining the process for maximum results.

So there it is.

So there lies the chicken sandwich right in front of you. The question is *simple.* Will you take back the helm of your ship and set a course that leads to a healthier you? Simply put, will you take back what is yours and OWN it?

Additional Thoughts

The Untapped Potential

As David and I worked through this book we talked about who this would impact. We talked about the millions of people who lead lives in an almost Zombie state. They wake up, go to work, come home and plop down in front of the TV or computer and zone out until it's time to go to bed.

I completely understand many people work two or three jobs or have kids to raise so it's difficult to find time to do anything, but exist. But what if you could carve out 30 minutes a day to make some kind of change. What if instead of sitting in front of the TV you picked up a book and read. What if reading 30 minutes a day was your minimum goal?

What if that translated to ten books over a year? I bet in those ten books you might find some nugget of knowledge or inspiration to work toward some improvement in your life or the lives of someone you love.

What if we could convince just 1% of the population to make positive changes in their lives and work toward improving the world around them? In the United States alone that would be an additional 330,000 people who are working to make themselves, their families or everyone around them better as a whole.

The untapped potential in this country is almost too vast to comprehend.

Ask most people today if a person can run a mile under 4 minutes and they will say, of course, but that wasn't always so. There was a time before 1954 that the "experts" thought it was physically impossible for a human to break that barrier. That was until Roger Bannister did it.

As striking as his feat was, what was even more striking is that the next year, FOUR more people ran a sub 4-minute mile. Three of them did it in a single race! What that tells us is that it only took one person, who's Self Image was that of a sub 4-minute miler. One person to show the rest of us what is possible. Those that followed in the next year saw themselves as already breaking that barrier because Roger validated its possibility and they did it. This kind of motivation comes from within.

Yes, competition can drive us to win, but even that comes from outside the individual. External motivation can temporarily get you off of the couch, but only until that external force goes away. Once the external force leaves you are back on the couch.

It is only by changing your SI that real, lasting change can occur and take hold.

"Can you lose internal motivation?"

Absolutely! That is why the good habit you take on must be reinforced on a daily basis. That is why I have often said, "Doing is to knowing as ten is to one." You can read all of the self-help books and listen to motivating podcasts, but until you put action to a goal it is simply a goal. One in which the world is poorer for because you chose not to fulfill it.

I have listened to many motivational tapes and read scores of books on the topic. I have even walked on red hot coals to show what is possible. These were all external forces. It wasn't until I started to work on my "inside game" that real and lasting change occurred.

Change can be scary, even small change. I have a mentor who has always told me, "feel the fear and do it anyway." So, I set my big audacious goals then break them down into ridiculously small movements. These movements are so embarrassingly small that I can't help but keep them and then just "DO." You can too. It is that easy. Don't make this harder than it needs to be. That is why we titled this book *The S.I.M.P.L.E. Plan.*

Don

About the Authors

David Havens was born and raised in Ohio. In 1987 he enlisted in the U.S. Navy as a Gunners Mate. His first command was the USS Richmond K. Turner CG-20, a Guided Missile Cruiser stationed in Charleston, SC. In 1991 he deployed to the Persian Gulf in support of Operation Desert Shield/Storm. In 1993 Dave attended Basic Underwater Demolition SEAL (BUD/S) training, graduating in BUD/S Class 190. David served 14 years in the SEAL Teams before retiring in 2008. During his career he made multiple deployments to Iraq in support of Operation Iraqi Freedom.

For the past 13 years David has been training and consulting various groups, in the Special Operations community, in the areas of Force Protection and Training Exercise Development.

Dave is also the author of three other books:

Front Sight Focus "Ten phrases US Navy SEALS use to ensure mission success." *Front Sight Focus* is a concept and mindset that is used by U.S. Navy

SEALs to plan and achieve success on and off of the battlefield as it reveals ten phrases that lead to efficiency at all levels of learning, training and productivity. Front Sight Focus is available on Amazon, Audible.com, Kindle and itunes.

Amphit For Life - The Workout System "A Common Sense Approach to Mission Planning Your Time in the Gym for Maximum Results" The Amphit For Life workout system teaches you how to plan a workout, rotate the exercises within the workout and calculate weight, sets and reps for each of the exercises. The workout and instructions are easy to follow and detailed enough for anyone from beginner to expert.

Bill and Dave's Daily Dose "*50 Posts to Motivate You to Elevate Your Life*" This book is a prescription for motivating you to elevate your *Life* and those around you. These daily doses are a combination of experiences as Chief Petty Officers in the U.S. Navy and some of our lessons learned from *Life.*

Donald Morris is a financial advisor and Certified Divorce Financial Analyst.

He served as Scoutmaster for a Boy Scout troop for almost ten years. An Eagle himself, he helped 27 youth achieve this coveted rank during his tenure.

He has backpacked a number of locations from the Adirondacks to the UP of Michigan to the Rocky Mountains.

He continues to look for his next great hiking adventure.

David Havens and Donald Morris are available for speaking engagements and individual coaching. For further information go to www.buckeyefrog.com or follow on Instagram @frontsightfocus190

Here is a list of books we recommend to assist you in your pursuit of Achievement:

Havens, David. *Front Sight Focus: Ten phrases U.S. Navy SEALs use to ensure mission success.* ETA Solutions LLC, 2016

Havens, David. *Bill & Dave's Daily Dose: 50 Posts To Motivate You To Elevate Your Life.* ETA Solutions LLC, 2018

Havens, David. *Amphit For Life: A Common Sense Approach to Mission Planning Your Time In The Gym For Maximum Results.* ETA Solutions LLC, 2020

Boothman, Nicholas. *How to Make People Like You in 90 Seconds or Less.* Workman Publishing Company, 2008

Guise, Stephen. *How to Be an Imperfectionist: The New Way to Self-Acceptance, Fearless Living, and*

Freedom from Perfectionism. Selective Entertainment LLC, 2015

Guise, Stephen. *Mini Habits: Smaller Habits, Bigger Results.* Selective Entertainment LLC, 2013

Hartwig, Dallas and Hartwig, Melissa. *It Starts with Food: Discover the Whole30 and Change Your Life in Unexpected Ways.* Victory Belt Publishing, 2014

Hill, Napoleon. *Think and Grow Rich.* Penguin Publishing Group, 2005

Walker, Matthew PhD. *Why We Sleep: Unlock The Power Of Sleep And Dreams.* Scribner, 2017

Willingham, Ron. *The Inner Game of Selling: Mastering the Hidden Forces that Determine Your Success.* Free Press, A Division of Simon & Schuster, Inc. 2006

Wyner, Gabriel. *Fluent Forever: How to Learn Any Language Fast and Never Forget It.* Harmony, 2014

Made in United States
Troutdale, OR
11/03/2026

56852550R00070